Table of Contents

Introduction 3
   Hemochromatosis 3
   Symptoms of hemochromatosis 4
   Causes of hemochromatosis 4
   Diagnosing hemochromatosis 6
   Hemochromatosis treatment 8
   Complications associated with hemochromatosis ... 9
   Lifestyle measures 10
Hemochromatosis Diet 11
   Dietary factors 11
   Foods to eat 12
   Foods to avoid 15
   Diet effect on this condition 18
Recipes #1 18
   Vegetable Quiche 18
   Turkey Chili 20
   Blueberry Salad with Grilled Turmeric Chicken 21
   Buttermilk Green Tea Roasted Chicken 25
   Split Pea and Mint Soup 28
   Baked Eggs in Avocado 32
   Linguine With Goat Cheese And Zucchini 36
   Vegetarian Club Sandwich With White Beans And Avocado 38

Soft Tacos With Mushrooms And Swiss Chard 39

Beefless Sloppy Joes 41

Recipes #2 43

Halibut With Citrus, Tomatoes, And Olives 43

Halibut With Sweet Potato And Lentils 44

Tuna With Mojo Sauce 46

Tuna Noodle Casserole 47

Grilled Snapper With Olives And White Wine Sauce 50

Lemon-Basil Spaghetti With Salmon 52

Coconut Fish Sticks With Yogurt Dipping Sauce 53

Seared Scallops With Mango Salsa 56

Salmon Burgers With Homemade Pickles 58

Shepherd's Pie 59

Classic Meatloaf With Ground Chicken 62

Introduction

Hemochromatosis causes the body to absorb too much iron from foods. By modifying their diet in specific ways, people with hemochromatosis can minimize the symptoms and reduce the risk of complications. There are two types of hemochromatosis: primary and secondary. Primary hemochromatosis is genetic, while secondary hemochromatosis can result from health conditions, such as liver disease and anemia. Most people absorb and lose about 1 milligram (mg) of iron per day. People with hemochromatosis can absorb up to 4 mg of iron each day. An excessive buildup of iron in the organs can be toxic and cause damage. However, it is possible to maintain healthy iron levels through dietary changes.

Hemochromatosis

Hemochromatosis is a medical condition in which too much iron builds up in the body. Serious health problems can arise because your body cannot eliminate the excess iron.

The excess iron builds up in your:

- liver
- skin

- heart
- pancreas
- joints
- pituitary gland

This buildup of iron can cause tissue and organ damage.

Symptoms of hemochromatosis

Many people with hemochromatosis don't have noticeable symptoms. When symptoms do exist, they may vary between individuals. Some common symptoms include:

- fatigue and weakness
- weight loss
- a low sex drive
- abdominal pain
- bronze or gray skin color
- joint pain

Causes of hemochromatosis

The two forms of hemochromatosis are primary and secondary.

Primary hemochromatosis

Primary hemochromatosis, also known as hereditary hemochromatosis, usually results from genetic factors.

The HFE gene, or hemochromatosis gene, controls how much iron you absorb from food. It lives on the short arm of chromosome 6. The two most common mutations of this gene are C28Y and H63D.

Usually, a person with hereditary hemochromatosis inherits a copy of the defective gene from each parent. However, not everyone who inherits the genes develops the illness. Researchers are looking into why some people have symptoms of iron overload and others do not.

In the United States, about 1 in 300 white, non-Hispanic people have this condition. Many do not realize they have it. Complications are more likely to occur in males and those with other medical problems like diabetes or liver disease.

In females, symptoms may not appear until after menopause. This is because menstruation tends to reduce iron levels in the blood. Once menstruation stops, levels may build up.

Secondary hemochromatosis

Secondary hemochromatosis occurs when a buildup of iron stems from another medical condition, such as erythropoietic hemochromatosis. In this disease, the red blood cells release too much iron into the body because they are too fragile.

Other risk factors for secondary hemochromatosis include:

alcohol dependency

a family history of diabetes, heart disease, or liver disease

taking iron or vitamin C supplements, which can increase the amount of iron the body absorbs

frequent blood transfusions

Diagnosing hemochromatosis
A doctor will:

- ask about symptoms

- ask about any supplements you may take

- ask about personal and family medical history

- carry out a physical exam

- recommend some tests

The symptoms can resemble those of many other conditions, making diagnosis difficult. Several tests may be necessary to confirm a diagnosis.

Blood testing

A blood test, such as a serum transferrin saturation (TS) test, can measure iron levels. A TS test measures how much iron is bound to the protein transferrin, which carries iron in your blood.

A blood test can also give an idea about your liver function.

Genetic testing

DNA testing can show if a person has genetic changes that may lead to hemochromatosis. If there is a family history of hemochromatosis, DNA testing can be useful for those planning to start a family.

For the test, a healthcare professional may draw blood or use a swab to collect cells from your mouth.

Liver biopsy

The liver is the main place where the body stores iron. It is usually one of the first organs damaged by iron buildup.

A liver biopsy can show if there is too much iron in the liver or if liver damage is present. The doctor will remove a small piece of tissue from your liver for testing in a lab.

MRI tests

MRI scans and other noninvasive tests can also measure iron levels in the body. A doctor may recommend an MRI test instead of a liver biopsy.

Hemochromatosis treatment

Treatment is available for managing high iron levels.

Phlebotomy

The main medical treatment is phlebotomy. This involves taking blood and iron from the body. A healthcare professional puts a needle into a vein, and blood flows into a bag, like when donating blood.

At first, around 1 pint of blood will be removed once or twice a week. When iron levels return to normal, you may need treatment every 2 to 4 months.

Chelation

Another option is chelation. This is a developing therapy that can help manage iron levels, but it is expensive and not a first-line treatment option.

A doctor may inject the drugs or give you pills. Chelation helps your body expel excess iron in your urine and stool.

However, there may be side effects, such as pain at the injection site and flu-like symptoms.

Chelation may be suitable for people with heart complications or other contraindications for phlebotomy.

Complications associated with hemochromatosis

Complications can arise in the organs that store excess iron. A person with hemochromatosis may have a higher risk of:

• liver damage, making a liver transplant necessary in some cases

• pancreatic damage, leading to diabetes

• joint damage and pain, such as arthritis

• heart problems, including irregular heartbeats and heart failure

• skin discoloration

- damage to the adrenal glands

- problems with the reproductive system, such as erectile dysfunction and menstrual irregularities

Early treatment and active management and monitoring of iron levels can help you avoid complications.

Lifestyle measures

Measures that can help you manage your health with hemochromatosis include:

- having annual blood tests to monitor iron levels

- avoiding multivitamins, vitamin C supplements, and iron supplements

- avoiding alcohol, which can cause additional damage to the liver

- taking care to avoid infections, for example, by having regular vaccinations and following good hygiene practices

- keeping a log of iron levels to monitor changes

- following all the doctor's instructions and attending all appointments

- contacting your doctor if symptoms worsen or change

- asking your doctor about counseling if symptoms affect your quality of life

Hemochromatosis Diet

Dietary factors

The goal of treating hemochromatosis is to reduce the amount of iron in the body to normal levels. As well as eating only foods that are low in iron, there are other factors to consider. For example, some dietary components affect how much iron the body absorbs.

Examples include:

Iron type: Heme iron is easier for the body to absorb than nonheme iron. Plant-based foods contain only nonheme iron, whereas meat, poultry, fish, and seafood contain both heme and nonheme iron.

Vitamin C: This vitamin enhances nonheme iron absorption.

Calcium: This mineral can reduce iron absorption.

Phytates, tannins, and polyphenols: These dietary components limit the absorption of nonheme iron.

In addition to dietary changes, doctors can treat hemochromatosis with medication and therapeutic phlebotomy, a treatment that removes blood from the body.

Foods to eat

There are no formal dietary guidelines for people with hemochromatosis, but some foods that may be beneficial include:

Fruits and vegetables

Fruits and vegetables are an important part of any healthful diet. They are rich in vitamins and minerals that are vital for the body to function properly.

Some fruits and vegetables, including spinach, mushrooms, and olives, are high in nonheme iron. As nonheme iron is harder for the body to absorb, they are unlikely to affect iron levels significantly.

People with hemochromatosis have higher levels of oxidative stress that can be damaging. Eating foods that contain antioxidants can counteract the oxidation and protect the cells from damage.

Many fruits and vegetables are high in antioxidants, such as vitamin E and selenium.

Plants also contain phytochemicals or plant compounds that provide protective properties. Examples of phytochemicals include:

- lutein in dark leafy greens
- lycopene in tomatoes
- anthocyanins in beets and blueberries

Lean protein

Lean protein is an essential part of a healthful, balanced diet, but many sources of lean protein contain iron.

Although there is no need for people with hemochromatosis to avoid animal protein completely, it is best to choose animal proteins that contain lower amounts of iron, such as fish and chicken, over iron-rich animal proteins, such as red meat.

Grains, beans, nuts, and seeds

All grains, legumes, seeds, and nuts contain phytic acid, or phytate, which reduces iron absorption.

Eating foods high in phytates, such as beans, nuts, and whole grains, reduces the absorption of nonheme iron from plant foods. As a result, it may reduce total iron levels in the body.

Tea and coffee

Tea and coffee contain tannins, which are types of polyphenol plant compounds.

The tannins in tea and coffee may reduce iron absorption. Drinking these beverages is another way for people with hemochromatosis to manage their iron levels.

Calcium-rich foods

Calcium can inhibit the absorption of both nonheme and heme iron.

Examples of calcium-rich foods include:

- yogurt
- milk
- cheese
- tofu
- green leafy vegetables, such as broccoli

Eggs

Research also suggests that eggs can help inhibit iron absorption.

Eggs contain a protein called phosvitin that binds to iron and prevents absorption.

Foods to avoid

Doctors generally advise people with hemochromatosis to avoid iron-fortified foods and supplements. Other foods to consider avoiding include:

Red meat

Most red meats, including beef, lamb, and venison, are a rich source of heme iron. Chicken and pork contain lower amounts of heme.

As heme iron is easy for the body to absorb, people with hemochromatosis may wish to avoid most red meat.

Red meat also enhances nonheme iron absorption.

Pairing red meat with foods that reduce iron absorption might also help control iron levels.

Raw shellfish

Shellfish, such as mussels, oysters, and clams, sometimes contain Vibrio vulnificus bacteria. These bacteria can cause a serious infection called vibriosis.

People with hemochromatosis are more susceptible to vibriosis infection. Therefore, it is important to cook any shellfish thoroughly to kill the bacteria. People can also reduce their risk of infection by discarding any raw shellfish that have open shells and avoiding eating any shellfish that remain unopened after cooking.

Vitamin C

Vitamin C increases the absorption of nonheme iron. Due to this, people with hemochromatosis should avoid vitamin C supplements.

The amount of vitamin C in fruits and vegetables is generally too low to have a significant effect on iron absorption. These foods also contain a variety of other nutrients that are important in a healthful diet.

However, eating foods or drinking beverages high in vitamin C alongside iron-rich foods may enhance iron absorption. For this reason, pairing iron-rich foods with vitamin C-rich foods may not be the best choice for those with hemochromatosis.

People should speak with a doctor to find out how much vitamin C they should be consuming each day.

Fortified foods

Fortified and enriched foods contain added vitamins and minerals to improve nutrition. Many cereal products are fortified with calcium, vitamin D, and iron.

People with hemochromatosis should avoid iron-fortified foods.

Alcohol

Digesting alcohol causes the body to produce substances that damage the liver.

Combining iron and alcohol can increase oxidative stress. This oxidative stress may worsen the effect of hemochromatosis on the body. Alcohol also increases the body's iron stores.

A doctor may suggest to a person with hemochromatosis that they limit their alcohol intake.

Diet effect on this condition

Diet can affect iron absorption, but whether it has much of an effect on hemochromatosis is unclear. Dietary changes could be unnecessary in people with hemochromatosis.

According to the American Association for the Study of Liver Diseases and the National Institute of Diabetes and Digestive and Kidney Diseases, dietary changes have only a small effect on iron levels compared with standard treatments for hemochromatosis. Although dietary changes may help reduce iron levels in small amounts, they are not nearly as effective as medications or phlebotomy.

However, the Centers for Disease Control and Prevention (CDC) and the National Heart, Lung, and Blood Institute still suggest that people with hemochromatosis should avoid:

- iron supplements
- vitamin C supplements
- raw shellfish
- high alcohol use

Recipes #1
Vegetable Quiche
Ingredients

- 1 tbsp. olive oil

- 1/2 cup green onion, chopped

- 1/2 cup onion, chopped

- 1/2 cup zucchini, chopped

- 1 cup spinach

- 3 eggs, beaten

- 1/2 cup milk

- 1 1/2 cups shredded cheese

- 1 deep dish pie crust, precooked

Directions

- Preheat the oven to 350°F (177°C).

- In a large skillet, heat the olive oil. Add the green onion, onion, and zucchini. Cook for 5 minutes.

- Add the spinach. Cook for an additional 2 minutes. Remove the cooked vegetables from the skillet and set aside.

- In a mixing bowl, whisk the eggs, milk, half of the cheese, and salt and pepper to taste.

- Pour the egg mixture into the pie crust. Top with the remainder of the shredded cheese.

- Bake for 40–45 minutes, or until the eggs are cooked throughout.

Turkey Chili

Ingredients

- 1 tbsp. olive oil

- 1 lb. ground turkey

- 1 large onion, chopped

- 2 cups chicken broth

- 1 (28-ounce) can red tomatoes, crushed

- 1 (16-ounce) can kidney beans, drained and rinsed

- 2 tbsp. chili powder

- 1 tbsp. garlic, chopped

- 1/2 tsp. each cayenne, paprika, dried oregano, cumin, salt, and pepper

Directions

- In a large pot over medium heat, heat olive oil. Add the ground turkey and cook until browned. Add the chopped onion and cook until tender.

- Add the chicken broth, tomatoes, and kidney beans. Add remaining ingredients and stir thoroughly.

- Bring to a boil then reduce heat to low. Cover and simmer for 30 minutes.

Blueberry Salad with Grilled Turmeric Chicken
Healthy Low-Iron Recipe

This fun mixture of flavors makes for a colorful salad: beautiful blueberries with fresh green lettuce, pure white cheese, and bright-orange grilled chicken.

The ingredients in this salad bring many tools for combating iron overload to the table: namely calcium and polyphenols.

Also significant is what this recipe does not include: it is naturally low in iron enhancers such as vitamin C or carotenoids and uses lower-iron ingredients such as chicken and butterhead lettuce (compared to higher iron options for protein and salad greens).

Why This Recipe Works for Hemochromatosis

CHICKEN:

When trying to eat a low-iron diet, animal meat is sometimes one of the first food groups to go. However, chicken tends to not be as high in iron as you might suspect, and meals made with chicken often make excellent options for lower-iron eating.

FETA OR BLUE CHEESE:

Calcium-rich dairy products like feta or blue cheese provide excellent blocking of both heme and non-heme iron from this entrée salad.

TURMERIC, CURRY POWDER, BLUEBERRIES, AND PECANS:

Turmeric, curry powder, blueberries, and pecans are all very rich in polyphenols. Polyphenols are health-promoting antioxidant nutrients that prevent iron from being absorbed from a meal. This recipe includes polyphenolic-rich foods in multiple places to boost their overall effects!

SALAD DRESSING:

Many salad dressings include acidic-ingredients such as vinegar, citrus juice, or soy sauce, all of which can enhance iron absorption and are contraindicated in low-iron recipes. This recipe utilizes the ingredients' natural flavors with a simple olive oil coating to maintain the flavor without accentuating iron absorption from the salad ingredients.

Ingredients

- 1 pound (450 g) chicken breasts, cut into 1-inch (2.5-cm) thick strips
- Salt and black pepper as needed
- 1 teaspoon ground turmeric
- ½ teaspoon curry powder
- 5 tablespoons (75 ml) olive oil, divided
- 4 cups (120 g) coarsely chopped butterhead lettuce
- 1 cup (144 g) fresh blueberries
- ½ cup (60 g) pecan halves
- 2 ounces (58 g) feta or blue cheese, crumbled

INSTRUCTIONS

- Season the chicken with the salt and pepper.

- In a small bowl, make a paste with the turmeric, curry powder, and 1 tablespoon (15 ml) of the oil. Coat the chicken strips in the paste and set them aside.

- Preheat the grill, electric grill, or stovetop grill pan to medium-high heat (400°F [200°C]). Spray it with cooking spray then add the chicken and cook 5 to 7 minutes per side (or 5 to 7 minutes total with a two-sided electric grill) until the chicken reaches an internal temperature of 165°F (74°C).

- Fill 4 salad bowls with the lettuce and coat it with the remaining 4 tablespoons (60 ml) oil, then top with the chicken strips, blueberries, pecans, and cheese.

NOTES

Why This Recipe Works for Hemochromatosis

- Maximum 1.6 mg iron per serving.

- Iron is blocked by the:

 - phytates in pecans;

 - polyphenols in turmeric, curry, blueberries and pecans;

 - calcium in cheese and pecans.

- Iron is not enhanced because:

- the vegetables recommended are low in vitamin C and carotenoids;

- this recipe does not use a vinegar-based salad dressing.

Buttermilk Green Tea Roasted Chicken
Healthy Low-Iron Recipe Featuring Chicken and Green Tea

When trying to eat a low-iron diet, animal meat is sometimes one of the first food groups eliminated. However, chicken tends to not be as high in iron as you might suspect, and meals made with chicken often make excellent options for lower-iron eating.

This easy week-night recipe starts with a classic technique (roasted chicken) and incorporates it with a delicious calcium and polyphenol-rich marinade to further limit iron absorption. Buttermilk is rich in calcium and makes a delicious marinade for chicken. The addition of green tea doesn't affect the taste—you'd never know it was in this meal!

Why This Recipe Works for Hemochromatosis

CHICKEN:

As lower-iron meat, this chicken dish only has 1.5 mg iron per 3-ounce (84-g) serving. Due to the addition of the calcium and polyphenol-rich ingredients used in this recipe, the total iron absorbed by your body will end up being even less!

BUTTERMILK:

Calcium-rich dairy products like buttermilk provide excellent blocking of both heme and non-heme iron from this chicken entrée.

GREEN TEA:

Green tea and the herbs thyme, sage, and rosemary, are all very rich in polyphenols. Polyphenols are health-promoting antioxidant nutrients that prevent iron from being absorbed from a meal.

MARINADE:

Most marinades will include acidic-ingredients such as vinegar, citrus juice, or soy sauce, all of which can enhance iron absorption and are contraindicated in low-iron recipes. This marinade preserves the tenderness and flavor of a traditional marinade without accentuating iron absorption from the meal. Win-win!

INGREDIENTS

- 1 teaspoon dried thyme
- 1 teaspoon dried sage
- 1 teaspoon ground mustard seeds
- 1 tablespoon (2 g) dried rosemary
- 2 teaspoons (10 g) salt
- 1 teaspoon ground black pepper
- 2 tablespoons (30 ml) honey
- 1 cup (240 ml) buttermilk
- 1 cup (240 ml) brewed green tea chilled
- 2 pounds (900 g) skin-on, bone-in chicken pieces (breasts, legs, and so on)

INSTRUCTIONS

- In a medium bowl, mix together the thyme, sage, mustard seeds, rosemary, salt, and pepper. Stir in the honey, buttermilk, and green tea. Place the chicken and the marinade in a large resealable bag or lidded bowl then refrigerate for at least 2 hours and up to 24 hours.

• Preheat the oven to 425°F (220°C). Line a medium roasting tray with foil. Let the excess marinade drip off the chicken pieces and place the pieces on the prepared roasting tray. Bake for approximately 30 minutes, until the chicken skin is crispy and the meat reaches an internal temperature of 165°F (74°C).

Split Pea and Mint Soup
Healthy Low-Iron Vegetarian and Vegan Recipe

This beautiful green soup, a vegetarian and vegan-friendly hemochromatosis recipe, is low in iron and rich in protein and phytates. This creamy soup makes for a great lunch or dinner for those looking for low-iron recipes. The mint brings a freshness to the overall flavor that is really pleasant!

You can make this into a vegan recipe by using non-dairy milk or by eliminating the milk altogether. Alternatively, if you're not a vegetarian, feel free to substitute the vegetable stock with chicken stock.

Why This Recipe Works for Hemochromatosis

SPLIT PEAS:

Legumes, such as split peas, are excellent sources of plant-based protein that are also rich in iron-blocking phytates. Some legumes may also be high in iron, but split peas are some of the lowest-iron legumes. When cooked correctly and combined intelligently, legumes become excellent options for an iron-reducing diet.

VEGETABLES:

A challenge when adding vegetables into a hemochromatosis recipe is to watch out that the vegetables themselves are not high in iron. It's also important to make sure they are not too high in iron-enhancers like vitamin C or carotenoids, which can cause the iron in the rest of the meal to be absorbed in greater amounts. Although green peas and onions both contain some of these nutrients, I have carefully adjusted the portions to keep their impact on iron absorption minimized so you can safely enjoy these healthy foods!

MILK:

Calcium-rich dairy products provide excellent blocking of both heme and non-heme iron. Non-dairy milk often contains calcium, too, so you are not limited to only cow's milk products.

GREEN TEA:

Green tea is very rich in polyphenols; polyphenols are health-promoting antioxidant nutrients that prevent iron from being absorbed from a meal.

INGREDIENTS

- ⅓ cup (66 g) dried green split peas

- 3½ cups (840 ml) water plus 1-2 Tbsp extra water

- 1 tablespoon (15 ml) extra virgin olive oil

- 2 medium onions coarsely chopped

- 3 cloves garlic minced

- 5 cups (1.2 L) vegetable stock

- ½ teaspoon salt plus more as needed

- ¼ teaspoon black pepper plus more as needed

- 2 green tea bags

- 10 ounces (280 g) fresh or frozen green peas

- 10 to 20 fresh mint leaves plus more as needed

- Milk or cream optional, to taste

INSTRUCTIONS

- Put the split peas and 3½ cups (840 ml) of the water in a large pot over high heat. Bring the split peas to a boil, then reduce the heat to medium and simmer, uncovered, for 30 to 40 minutes, until the split peas are tender and most of the water is absorbed. Scoop the cooked split peas from the pot into a small bowl.

- In the same large pot over medium heat, combine oil, onions, and additional 1 to 2 tablespoons (15 to 30 ml) water. Cook the onions for 5 minutes, then add the garlic and cook 2 additional minutes, stirring frequently.

- Add the split peas, vegetable stock, salt, and pepper and bring the mixture to a boil over high heat. Reduce the heat to medium, add the green tea bags, stir, and simmer, uncovered, for 5 minutes.

- Add the green peas and mint, and adjust the temperature as needed to keep the soup at a gentle simmer for 10 to 15 minutes.

- Remove the pot from the heat, remove and discard the green tea bags, and let the soup cool for 10 minutes.

- Puree the soup using a blender or immersion blender. Season the soup with additional salt, pepper, and/or mint to taste. Add the milk (if using) to make a creamy soup.

- Serve the soup garnished with an additional mint leaf.

NOTES

- Use nondairy milk to make this soup vegan.

- If you aren't vegetarian, chicken stock will also work well in this recipe.

- For a thicker soup, simmer longer to reduce the liquid to your desired consistency.

Baked Eggs in Avocado
Healthy Low-Iron Breakfast Recipe

Breakfast can be a challenging meal when you learn you have hemochromatosis. A reader once wrote to us, "I need breakfast ideas as most of the cereals I used to eat I found out were iron-fortified!"

Breakfast foods are also often heavy in iron-rich meats and may be served with vitamin C–rich fruit or fruit juices, adding to the frustration.

Thankfully, many traditional breakfast foods can still be incorporated into a hemochromatosis diet.

Why This Recipe Works for Hemochromatosis

EGGS:

In the world of hemochromatosis, if you like or can eat eggs, they can quickly become one of your best friends. They can be an excellent source of dietary protein that doesn't increase iron levels.

At first glance, eggs seem to be high in iron. One large chicken egg contains just shy of 1 mg of iron. But eggs also contain something called phosvitin, the "egg factor" that blocks iron not only from the egg itself but also from the rest of the meal. The more eggs you eat at one sitting, the more iron that's blocked from that meal! Studies have shown that adding three eggs to a meal may reduce iron absorption by nearly 80 percent.*

AVOCADO:

A nutrient-dense fruit (yes, it's a fruit, not a vegetable!), avocado is full of good fats, naturally low in sugar and salt, and delicious. The good news for you is that it's also naturally low in iron!

CURRY POWDER:

Curry powder is just one of many herbs and spices high in polyphenols, health-promoting antioxidant nutrients also prevent iron from being absorbed from a meal.

INGREDIENTS

- 1 large avocado
- Salt and black pepper to taste
- Curry powder to taste (optional)
- 2 large eggs
- 1 tablespoon (3 g) fresh cilantro finely chopped
- Olive oil to taste

INSTRUCTIONS

- Preheat the oven to 425°F (220°C).

- Slice the avocado in half and remove the pit. Slice a small section from the back of each half to make a flat surface in the skin, then place both halves, flesh-side up, on a small rimmed baking sheet lined with foil. Using a spoon, carefully scoop out some of the flesh to make a little more space for the eggs but don't go all the way to the skin. Place the scooped-out avocado flesh in a medium bowl and set aside.

- Sprinkle the salt and pepper and curry powder (if using) on both avocado halves. Carefully break an egg into each half, being sure not to break the yolks. Sprinkle some additional salt and pepper and curry powder (if using) on the eggs if desired.

- Bake the avocado halves for 15 minutes for a poached egg (with a runny yolk), or 18 to 20 minutes if you prefer your eggs more solid.

- While the eggs are baking, add salt, the cilantro, and olive oil to the reserved avocado. Mash lightly to make a topping for the eggs.

- Once the eggs are done, remove them from the oven and let them sit 1 minute. Place each avocado half in a bowl.

Scrape up any crispy eggs that remain on the baking sheet and add them to each bowl for an extra crunch. Top the eggs with the avocado-herb mixture and eat with a spoon.

NOTES

• If you've ever cut open an avocado only to realize it was too hard and not ripe yet, this is a great way to salvage it. After being baked, the avocado will end up perfectly soft, no matter how it starts out.

• Don't be tempted to skip lining the baking sheet with foil; this recipe can create a very stubborn baked-on mess that takes a lot of elbow grease to clean. Trust me on this one.

Linguine With Goat Cheese And Zucchini

Goat cheese is lower in fat and calories than many hard cheeses. And because it's so soft, it melts beautifully into a creamy sauce, like in this pasta dish.

Ingredients

- 12 ounces whole-wheat linguine

- 1 tablespoon extra-virgin olive oil

- 1 pound zucchini, cut into thin half-moons

- 1¼ teaspoons salt

- ½ teaspoon freshly ground black pepper

- 1 garlic clove, chopped

- 5 ounces goat cheese

- 2 teaspoons grated lemon zest

Directions

- Cook the linguine according to the package directions. Drain the pasta, reserving 1 cup of the pasta water, and return the linguine to the pot.

- Meanwhile, heat the oil in a medium skillet over medium-high heat. Add the zucchini, ½ teaspoon of salt, and ¼ teaspoon of pepper. Cook, stirring, until the zucchini is tender and any liquid has evaporated, about 5 minutes.

- Stir in the garlic and cook for 1 minute.

- Add all but 2 tablespoons of the cheese to the linguine in the pot. Add the reserved pasta water, the remaining ¾ teaspoon of salt, and the remaining ¼ teaspoon of pepper to the linguine. Stir until creamy.

- Serve the linguine topped with the zucchini, lemon zest, and the remaining 2 tablespoons of cheese.

Vegetarian Club Sandwich With White Beans And Avocado

Club sandwiches usually contain bacon, mayonnaise, and other meats and cheese—not ideal for someone on a low-cholesterol diet. This version is as satisfying as the real thing but uses creamy white beans as a spread and lots of vegetables for crunch.

Ingredients

- two 15-ounce cans of white beans, rinsed and drained
- 2 tablespoons extra-virgin olive oil
- ½ teaspoon salt
- ¼ teaspoon black freshly ground pepper
- 12 slices multigrain bread
- 1 red onion, thinly sliced
- 1 cucumber, thinly sliced
- one 4-ounce container sprouts (alfalfa, radish, broccoli, or any mix)

- 2 avocados,

- peeled, pitted, and thinly sliced

Directions

- In a medium bowl, combine the beans, oil, salt, and pepper. Mash the beans with a fork.

- Place 8 slices of bread on a work surface. Divide the mashed beans among them; top each with the onion, cucumber, sprouts, and avocado.

- Stack one open-faced sandwich on top of another until you have four double-decker sandwiches. Top each sandwich with remaining 4 slices of bread; plate and enjoy.

Soft Tacos With Mushrooms And Swiss Chard

Mushrooms, greens, and beans make a healthful, nutritious filling for corn tortillas. Opt for soft tortillas over crispy shells to save on fat and calories.

Ingredients

- ½ cup water

- 2 yellow onions, thinly sliced

- 1 teaspoon reduced-sodium tamari

- 8 ounces sliced button mushrooms

- 1 bunch swiss chard, stems and leaves separated and both thinly sliced

- one 15-ounce can pinto beans, rinsed and drained

- 8 corn tortillas

- 1 red bell pepper, seeded and chopped

Directions

- Bring the water to a simmer in a deep skillet over medium-high heat. Add the onions and cook for 8 minutes, stirring occasionally, until they begin to soften and brown.

- Add the tamari, mushrooms, and Swiss chard stems and reduce the heat to medium. Cover and cook for 15 minutes or until the mushrooms are tender, stirring frequently and adding 1 or 2 tablespoons of water if the onions begin to stick.

- Stir in the Swiss chard leaves and beans, cover, and cook for 5 minutes or until the leaves wilt.

- Warm the tortillas, fill them with the bean mixture, and serve topped with the red bell pepper.

Beefless Sloppy Joes

Sloppy Joe sandwiches are traditionally made with ground beef, which may make them high in saturated fat. This version substitutes mushrooms instead, meaning you get all the flavor without harming your heart.

Ingredients

- 1 pound cremini mushrooms, halved
- 1 tablespoon extra-virgin olive oil
- 1 large sweet onion, diced
- 1½ cups plus 4 tablespoons light beer
- ¼ teaspoon salt, plus more for seasoning
- ⅓ cup finely chopped walnuts
- 1 green pepper, diced
- ¾ teaspoon freshly ground black pepper
- ½ teaspoon chipotle chili powder
- ¼ cup ketchup
- 3 tablespoons tomato paste
- 6 whole-wheat hamburger buns

Directions

• Pulse the mushrooms in batches in a food processor until they are finely chopped.

• Heat the oil in a large nonstick skillet over medium-high heat. Add the onion, 1 tablespoon of the beer, and salt, and cook, stirring frequently, until the onion is lightly browned, about 5 minutes.

• Add the walnuts and green pepper, and cook, stirring occasionally, for 3 minutes.

• Add the mushrooms, black pepper, and chipotle chili powder. Cook, stirring frequently, for about 5 minutes or until mushrooms are just cooked through.

• Add the remaining beer, the ketchup, tomato paste, and a large pinch of salt. Cook while stirring until the sauce is a fairly thick consistency, about 2 minutes.

• Spoon the mixture onto the buns and serve.

Recipes #2

Halibut With Citrus, Tomatoes, And Olives

Halibut has a sweeter flavor than other fish, and firm, white flesh. If you can't find it in the seafood section, cod and haddock will both work well.

Ingredients

- 1 tablespoon extra-virgin olive oil, divided

- 1 yellow onion, thinly sliced

- 1 cup green olives, pitted and halved

- 2 oranges, peeled, separated into segments, and membranes removed

- one 28-ounce can diced tomatoes, undrained

- ¼ teaspoon salt

- ¼ teaspoon black pepper

- 1½ pounds halibut, skin removed, cut into 2-inch pieces

- ¼ cup fresh dill, chopped

Directions

- Heat the oil in a large saucepan over medium heat. Add the onion and cook until it is soft, about 5 minutes.

- Add the olives, orange segments, and tomatoes. Cover and simmer for 10 minutes. Add the salt and pepper.

- Place the fish in the pan and spoon the sauce over it. Cover and simmer until the fish is cooked through, about 7 minutes.

- Divide the fish and sauce among four plates, sprinkle with dill, and serve.

Halibut With Sweet Potato And Lentils

Lentils, rich in folic acid, fiber, and vitamins, belong in everyone's diet, and they are also an economical source of protein without cholesterol. Their different varieties—brown, green, and red—are relatively interchangeable, although brown and red lentils have a shorter cooking time.

Ingredients

- 2 tablespoons extra-virgin olive oil, divided

- 1 onion, chopped

- 2 garlic cloves, chopped

- 1 sweet potato, peeled and cut into ¼-inch pieces

- 2½ cups low-sodium chicken broth

- 1¼ cups green lentils, rinsed

- Salt and freshly ground black pepper

- Four 6-ounce pieces of halibut fillet

- ¼ cup dijon mustard

- ¼ cup dry white wine

- 1 tablespoon chopped fresh tarragon

Directions

- Heat 1 tablespoon of the olive oil in a large saucepan over medium heat. Add the onion and cook, stirring occasionally, until soft, 5 to 6 minutes.

- Add the garlic and sweet potato, and cook, stirring, for 1 minute.

- Add the broth and lentils, and simmer, covered, until lentils are tender, 20 to 25 minutes. Season with salt and pepper.

- Meanwhile, heat the remaining tablespoon of oil in a skillet over medium high heat. Season the fish with salt and pepper and cook in the skillet until opaque throughout, 3 to 5 minutes per side.

- In a small bowl, whisk together the mustard, wine, and tarragon.

- Serve the fish over the lentils and drizzled with the sauce.

Tuna With Mojo Sauce

Mojo is a citrus-based sauce made with garlic, olive oil, and fresh herbs. It goes perfectly with tuna steaks, which may be served medium-rare. To cook them medium-well done, increase the grilling time to four to six minutes per side.

Ingredients

- 4 garlic cloves, chopped

- 5 tablespoons extra-virgin olive oil

- 1 fresh jalapeño, seeded and thinly sliced

- Juice of 4 limes

- ⅓ cup fresh cilantro, coarsely chopped

- 1 teaspoon salt, plus more for seasoning

- Freshly ground black pepper

- Two 12-ounce tuna steaks, about 1¼-inch thick

Directions

- Heat an outdoor grill or indoor grill pan to medium-high.

- In a medium microwave-safe bowl, stir together the garlic and 4 tablespoons of olive oil. Cover it loosely with plastic wrap and microwave it until the garlic is soft and aromatic, about 2 minutes.

- Stir in the jalapeño, lime juice, cilantro, and salt. Set aside to cool.

- Brush the tuna with the remaining tablespoon of olive oil and season with salt and pepper.

- Grill the tuna, turning once, until the fish has grill marks on its surface, 3 to 5 minutes per side for medium rare. Let rest for 5 minutes.

- Slice each tuna steak in half and serve drizzled with the mojo.

Tuna Noodle Casserole

This dish is often made with egg noodles and high-fat cream of mushroom soup. While delicious, it isn't necessarily heart-healthful. This recipe does things differently by using fresh mushrooms, 2 percent milk, broccoli, and whole-wheat noodles.

Ingredients

- ½ pound whole-wheat fettuccine, broken into thirds
- 5 slices whole-wheat bread
- 1 tablespoon organic canola oil
- 1 cup chopped onion
- 1 celery stalk, finely diced
- one 10-ounce box white mushrooms, stemmed and chopped
- ¼ cup flour
- 3 cups 2 percent milk
- 1 cup low-sodium chicken broth
- ¼ teaspoon ground black pepper
- one 10-ounce box frozen chopped broccoli, thawed
- one 10-ounce box frozen peas, thawed
- four 6-ounce cans chunk light tuna in water, drained

Directions

• Preheat the oven to 425°F.

• Bring a pot of water to a boil and cook the fettuccine according to the package directions. Drain and set aside.

• Place the bread in a food processor and pulse for 30 seconds until it becomes breadcrumbs.

• Heat the oil in a large skillet over medium heat. Add the onion and cook, stirring, until translucent, about 5 minutes.

• Add the celery and cook, stirring, until just tender, about 6 minutes.

• Add the mushrooms and cook, stirring, until they release their liquid, 5 to 7 minutes.

• Add the flour and stir vigorously with a wooden spoon until there are no lumps.

• Add the milk and broth, stir to combine, and bring the mixture to a boil, stirring frequently.

• Reduce the heat to a vigorous simmer and cook, stirring, until the liquid thickens and reduces by about ½ cup, 7 to 8 minutes.

- Add the pepper and stir to combine.

- In a large bowl, combine the fettuccine, vegetable and mushroom mixture, broccoli, peas, and tuna.

- Pour the ingredients into a 9-by-13-inch casserole. Top with the breadcrumbs and bake for 25 minutes or until the top is golden and toasted. Serve hot.

Grilled Snapper With Olives And White Wine Sauce

When choosing a white wine for this dish, a dry white is best, such as Sauvignon Blanc, Chardonnay, or Pinot Grigio.

Ingredients

- four 6-ounce snapper fillets

- 2 tablespoons extra-virgin olive oil, plus more for the fish

- salt and freshly ground black pepper

- 1 onion, finely sliced

- 2 garlic cloves, finely chopped

- ¼ cup dry white wine

- 2 tomatoes, chopped

- ¼ cup green olives, pitted and chopped

- 2 tablespoons capers

- 1 serrano pepper, finely chopped

- ½ teaspoon sugar

- 1 bay leaf

Directions

- Heat the grill to high.

- Brush the snapper with some oil and season with salt and pepper. Grill for 2 minutes per side, remove from the grill, and cover to keep warm.

- Heat the oil in a medium skillet over medium-high heat. Add the onions and garlic, and cook until soft, 5 to 7 minutes.

- Add the wine and cook for 3 to 5 minutes or until slightly reduced.

- Add the tomatoes, olives, capers, serrano pepper, sugar, and bay leaf. Bring the sauce to a boil and cook until thickened.

- Reduce the heat, add the fish, and cook for 2 minutes or until the fish is completely cooked through.

- Spoon the fish fillets onto four plates and serve each with the olives and sauce.

Lemon-Basil Spaghetti With Salmon

Like tuna, salmon is another fish that may be served successfully anywhere between medium-rare to well-done. If you like salmon medium rare, cook it for two minutes per side.

Ingredients

- ½ pound whole-wheat spaghetti 1 garlic clove, minced

- 3 tablespoons extra-virgin olive oil

- ½ teaspoon salt, plus more for seasoning

- ½ teaspoon freshly ground black pepper, plus more for seasoning

- four 4-ounce salmon fillets

- ¼ cup chopped fresh basil leaves

- 3 tablespoons capers

- zest of 1 lemon

- 2 tablespoons lemon juice

- 2 cups baby spinach

Directions

- Bring a large pot of water to a boil. Add the spaghetti and cook, stirring occasionally, 8 to 10 minutes. Drain and transfer the spaghetti to a large bowl.

- Add the garlic, 2 tablespoons of olive oil, ½ teaspoon of salt, and ½ teaspoon of pepper, and toss to combine.

- Heat the remaining tablespoon of olive oil in a medium skillet over medium-high heat.

- Season the salmon fillets with salt and pepper, and cook them to the desired degree of doneness. Remove the salmon from the pan.

- Add the basil, capers, lemon zest, and lemon juice to the spaghetti and toss to combine.

- Place ½ cup of spinach each into four shallow bowls. Divide the spaghetti among the bowls and serve topped with a piece of salmon.

Coconut Fish Sticks With Yogurt Dipping Sauce

This kid-friendly recipe makes eating fish fun by coating it in a crunchy coconut-breadcrumb mixture. The fish sticks may also be frozen on a baking sheet uncooked and stored for up to one month in the freezer. Bake them directly from the freezer for 20 to 25 minutes.

Ingredients

For the fish sticks:

- cooking spray
- 1½ pounds tilapia fillets
- 1¼ cups whole-wheat breadcrumbs
- ⅓ cup sweetened shredded coconut
- 2 tablespoons yellow cornmeal
- 1 teaspoon mild curry powder
- ½ teaspoon salt, plus more for seasoning
- 1 free-range or omega-3 egg white
- 1 tablespoon water

For the yogurt dipping sauce:

- ⅓ cup 2 percent greek yogurt
- 1 carrot, peeled and finely grated

- 2 teaspoons sweet chili sauce

- 1 teaspoon low-sodium soy sauce

- 1 scallion, finely chopped

- juice of ½ lime

- 1 tablespoon water

Directions

To make the fish sticks:

- Preheat the oven to 425°F.

- Place a baking rack in a baking pan and spray it with cooking spray.

- Cut the fish into sticks about 3 inches long and ½-inch thick.

- In a food processor, combine the breadcrumbs, coconut, cornmeal, curry powder, and salt. Pulse until the coconut is coarsely chopped. Transfer the mixture to a shallow dish.

- In a separate shallow dish, whisk together the egg white and water.

- Dip each fish stick first into the egg white, shaking off the excess, and then coat each fish stick thoroughly with the breadcrumb mixture.

- Spray the fish sticks with cooking spray, arrange them on the baking rack, and bake them for 15 to 20 minutes, turning them halfway through. Bake them until golden, crispy, and cooked through. Season with salt.

To make the yogurt dipping sauce:

- Combine the yogurt, carrot, chili sauce, soy sauce, scallion, lime juice, and water in a medium bowl. Season with salt.

- Cover and refrigerate until serving. Serve alongside the hot fish sticks.

Seared Scallops With Mango Salsa

This recipe calls for sea scallops, which are larger than bay scallops and are readily available in the supermarket. You might notice a little muscle attached to the scallops. It hangs off to the side like a tag and you can remove it with your fingers.

Ingredients

- 1 cup brown rice

- 2 mangoes, pitted and cut into ½-inch pieces
- 1 cucumber, peeled and cut into ½-inch pieces
- 1 tablespoon grated fresh ginger
- 2 teaspoons fresh lime juice
- 2 tablespoons extra-virgin olive oil
- ½ cup fresh cilantro, chopped
- ½ teaspoon salt, plus more for seasoning
- freshly ground black pepper
- 1½ pounds sea scallops

Directions

- Cook the rice according to the package directions.

- In a medium bowl, combine the mangoes, cucumber, ginger, lime juice, 1 tablespoon of olive oil, cilantro, ½ teaspoon of salt, and a large pinch of pepper.

- Rinse the scallops and pat dry with paper towels. Season them with salt and pepper.

- Heat the remaining tablespoon of oil in a large skillet over medium-high heat. Add the scallops and cook until cooked through and golden brown, about 2 minutes per side.

- Serve with the rice and top with salsa.

Salmon Burgers With Homemade Pickles

This recipe uses raw salmon but if you use canned salmon, the dish is ready in a jiffy because the patties won't have to be completely cooked, only heated through.

Ingredients

- ¼ cup rice vinegar

- 1 tablespoon sugar

- ¾ teaspoon salt,

- 1 kirby cucumber, very thinly sliced

- ¼ white onion, thinly sliced

- 1¼ pounds skinless salmon fillet, cut into 1-inch pieces

- 4 scallions, thinly sliced

- ¼ teaspoon freshly ground black pepper

- 4 whole-wheat hamburger buns

Directions

• In a medium bowl, combine the vinegar, sugar, and ¼ teaspoon of salt, stirring until everything is dissolved.

• Add the cucumber and onion, and toss to combine. Let sit, tossing occasionally, for at least 15 minutes and up to 6 hours.

• Heat the grill to medium-high.

• In a food processor, pulse the salmon 3 or 4 times just until coarsely chopped.

• Add the scallions, the remaining ½ teaspoon of salt, and pepper, and pulse to combine.

• Form the mixture into four ¾-inch-thick patties.

• Oil the grill grate. Grill the patties, turning once, until opaque, 2 to 4 minutes per side.

• To serve, place the burgers on buns and top them with the cucumber and onion.

Shepherd's Pie

Shepherd's pie is one of the classic comfort foods that makes a perfect dinner on a cold winter day. It is usually made with ground beef, but this is a lighter version with ground turkey. And because it calls for red skinned potatoes, there is no need to peel them.

Ingredients

- 1 tablespoon extra-virgin olive oil
- 2 garlic cloves, minced
- 1 carrot, peeled and finely diced
- 1 onion, chopped
- 8 ounces ground turkey
- ½ teaspoon finely chopped fresh thyme
- 2 tablespoons ketchup
- 1 cup low-sodium chicken broth
- 2 teaspoons flour
- ½ cup frozen peas, thawed
- ¼ teaspoon salt, plus more for seasoning
- 1 pound red-skinned potatoes, cubed
- ½ cup 2 percent milk, warmed

- ⅓ cup shredded sharp cheddar cheese

- 1 scallion, chopped

- freshly ground black pepper

- cooking spray

Directions

- Preheat the oven to 425°F.

- Heat the oil in a medium ovenproof skillet over medium-high heat. Add the garlic, carrot, and onion. Cook until they are tender and begin to brown, about 5 minutes.

- Add the turkey and thyme, and cook, breaking the turkey up with a spoon, until it is cooked through and lightly browned.

- Stir in the ketchup and cook for 1 minute.

- In a small bowl, stir the broth and flour together until smooth. Pour the mixture into the skillet and cook until it thickens, about 2 minutes. Stir the peas in and add the salt.

- Meanwhile, place the potatoes in a medium pot and cover with water. Bring to a boil, lower the heat, and simmer until the potatoes are tender.

- Drain the potatoes and return them to the pot over low heat. Stir for 2 to 3 minutes to dry them out. Add the milk, cheese, and scallion, and mash the potatoes. Season with salt and pepper.

- Spoon the mashed potatoes over the meat filling and spread it in an even layer.

- Lightly mist the potatoes with nonstick cooking spray and bake until they are lightly browned and the filling is bubbling around the edges, 10 to 15 minutes. Serve hot.

Classic Meatloaf With Ground Chicken

All the flavors of traditional meatloaf are here but with a leaner meat than ground beef. Serve with mashed potatoes or roasted veggies and you have the perfect weeknight dinner.

Ingredients

- 1-pound ground chicken

- ½ cup fine breadcrumbs

- 1 free-range or omega-3 egg white

- 1 carrot, peeled and cut into chunks

- 1 onion, cut into chunks

- ¼ cup ketchup

- ½ teaspoon minced garlic

- 1 teaspoon worcestershire sauce

- ¼ teaspoon celery seed

- 1 teaspoon salt

- pinch of pepper

Directions

- Preheat the oven to 350°F.

- In a large bowl, combine the chicken, breadcrumbs, and egg white.

- In a blender combine the carrot, onion, ketchup, garlic, Worcestershire sauce, celery seed, salt, and pepper. Process until the carrot is very fine.

- Add the vegetable mixture to the meat and mix well with your hands.

- Form the mixture into a loaf and place it in a lightly greased 9-by-13-inch pan. Cover the loaf with foil and bake for 1 hour.

- Remove the foil and continue baking the loaf for 15 to 30 minutes, or until meatloaf is cooked through.

- Slice the loaf into 8 pieces and serve hot.

Made in the USA
Las Vegas, NV
09 September 2022